Group-Based Interventions for 'Understanding Brain Injury'

This hands-on volume is both manual and workbook, designed to be used alongside the Understanding Brain Injury Group. This group aims to increase the understanding and acknowledgement of acquired brain injury and find ways of coping with the consequences. The manual section outlines the steps needed for practitioners to run the Understanding Brain Injury Group successfully, and the workbook section – also available as a downloadable resource – is intended to be used by patients.

The chapters in the manual mirror the structure of the eight sessions of the group, highlighting differing aspects of having a brain injury. Initially, the sessions cover psychoeducation regarding brain injury and what neurorehabilitation entails. Following this, the group then focuses on living with the consequences of brain injury, whether that represents physical, cognitive, emotional or lifestyle changes. Participants are invited to share their experiences and discuss coping strategies to help with both the new limitations as well as the unwanted emotions that frequently exist after brain injury. Goals are set at the beginning of the group and are revisited at the end to decide on whether they were being realistic, overachieving or pessimistic in their outlook at the start of the group. Throughout, the members of the group can record their session activity in the accompanying workbook.

Created to be used by clinicians, therapists or any individual, this resource can be used in a post-acute setting such as a neurorehabilitation unit, a slow-stream rehab setting such as community neurorehabilitation or homes specifically aimed at catering for the needs of those with neurological impairments.

Dr Rebekah Jamieson-Craig is a qualified Clinical Psychologist from University College London, UK, and is currently employed by Barts Health NHS Trust. Throughout her career, she has had an interest in neurological conditions, and has worked within a brain injury neurorehabilitation unit, as well as several other neurorehabilitation settings.

T0383718

Group-Based Interventions for 'Understanding Brain Injury'

A Manual and Workbook for Practitioners and Patients

Rebekah Jamieson-Craig

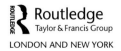

Routledge
Taylor & Francis Group

LONDON AND NEW YORK

Cover image: © Getty Images

First published 2024
by Routledge
4 Park Square, Milton Park, Abingdon, Oxon OX14 4RN

and by Routledge
605 Third Avenue, New York, NY 10158

Routledge is an imprint of the Taylor & Francis Group, an informa business

British Library Cataloguing-in-Publication Data
A catalogue record for this book is available from the British Library

ISBN: 978-1-032-57952-8 (hbk)
ISBN: 978-1-032-57951-1 (pbk)
ISBN: 978-1-003-44178-6 (ebk)

DOI: 10.4324/9781003441786

Typeset in Optima
by KnowledgeWorks Global Ltd.

Access the Support Material: www.routledge.com/9781032579511

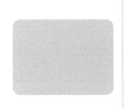

Contents

Acknowledgements

With thanks to Dr Tarick Ali, Clinical Psychologist, who helped me conceptualise how to create the 'Understanding Brain Injury' Group.

Also thanks to the many Trainee Clinical Psychologists and Assistant Psychologists, without whom the group would not have run as successfully for so many years.

Why create this manual?

Rehabilitation of those who have acquired a brain injury is a worldwide issue. Currently brain injury is one of the leading causes of death and disability worldwide (WHO, 2019). As of 2019, there were approximately 1.3 million people living with the consequences of brain injury in the UK alone (House of Commons, Acquired Brain Injury Debate pack, 2019). It is estimated by the charity Headway that a brain injury occurs every 90 seconds in the UK (2020). In the United States of America, it is estimated that 5.3 million people are living with the long-term consequences of traumatic brain injury. With these figures in mind, rehabilitating survivors of brain injury, so that they may be able to participate in everyday life, becomes imperative.

This manual is created to help anyone, regardless of their profession, who wishes to run an Understanding Brain Injury Group. It gives the facilitators ideas on how I ran many successful groups over a number of years. It is to be used in conjunction with the Understanding Brain Injury workbook. Without the manual, the workbook would seem somewhat like didactic teaching – which is most definitely not the purpose of this group. Rather, it is to be an interactive group, in which all members tell their own stories and describe the difficulties they are experiencing since their brain injury.

This manual outlines how to run an Understanding Brain Injury Group for those who have experienced any form of brain injury. It can, and has been, tailored to more specific conditions, such as stroke or how to manage after a cardiac event, as well as for working with family members of those who have experienced a brain injury.

DOI: 10.4324/9781003441786-1

This group comprises eight sessions; in this manual, I go through each session individually, outlining it and giving ideas for prompting questions that can be asked of the group to elicit discussion about their brain injury, how they feel emotionally and what coping strategies they have encountered and found helpful.

2 Introducing the group

The Understanding Brain Injury Group, or UBI for short, is a group designed to increase the individual's insight into the cause and effects of their brain injury. Although this was the primary function of the group initially, after many redevelopments, it is now only part of the purpose. Other objectives of the group include helping the individual with the brain injury identify the changes and difficulties the brain injury has caused, how they feel about these difficulties and what they can do to help cope with them. In short, this group is now just as much about giving individuals space to discover that they are not alone in suffering from a brain injury, to learn from each other's experiences and to discover new ways of coping with the challenges of surviving a brain injury, as it is about gaining insight into how their brain injury will affect them in their future.

The group is divided into eight sessions, each of which will be covered in more detail later in this manual. Before starting the group, however, some factors should be considered. For example, how many facilitators are needed to run the group? What size should the group be? How long should each session be? What about the group mix – gender, age, disability? Are there any reasons to exclude someone from the group? Each of these questions is valid, and although I can't tell you what would definitively be best, I can tell you what I have found to help over the years that I have run this group.

Facilitators

There are no hard and fast rules over which profession should run this group, but it is important that whoever facilitates it knows the individual members well. Even though it is possible to run this group on your own, it is helpful if

DOI: 10.4324/9781003441786-2

there are two people to co-facilitate. Generally, one person would lead the group, asking the questions and importing information where appropriate, whilst the other person aids by writing the suggestions made by the group on the flip-chart, checking that no one is being left out and enabling the participants to complete the workbook. Often, my co-facilitator and I would switch roles each session, so that the group could benefit from the slightly different styles each person has when running a group.

Size

In my experience, the ideal number of participants is somewhere between four and six. Initially, I tried running larger groups than this; however, there would always be at least one person who would get 'lost' during the group. It can be quite difficult to facilitate the group and make sure all the members are getting a chance to get their point across. This would be the case in any large group, but especially becomes the case when working with people with neurological disabilities, as often the individuals will have slower pro-cessing speeds, may have speech difficulties or just be shy within the group setting. With smaller groups, it is far more feasible to make sure that every-one who wishes to speak is given ample space and time to do so. Another consideration to be made regarding group size is that smaller groups can then take place in more relaxed settings; when running a group of eight, I would have to use the formal meeting room, where often the group dynam-ics were lost, ending up more as if I were the teacher and the members my students, who would contribute occasionally. However, when the group was a smaller size, it was possible to use a smaller therapy room, where all members sat around a circular table with the flip-chart in the corner of the room. This immediately created a more intimate setting, which in turn resulted in the members feeling more comfortable sharing their opinions and experiences with each other.

Length

I generally gave myself an hour to an hour-and-a-half to complete each UBI session. This included the time it would take to ready the participants – as I ran this group in an in-patient setting, this often involved going to the participants room and reminding them that it was time for the group. This would often take up to 15 minutes at the start of each session. Given this, each group session can easily be accomplished within an hour. It can be useful to have a little extra time during the sessions to specifically look at the difficulties caused by brain injury, as I discovered the members of the group would frequently become wrapped up in discussing what they now found challenging. A further point is the frequency of the group. Again, this is up to the facilitator, but I found it helpful to run two sessions a week when possible; this way the members did not have too long of a gap between the sessions, so less information would be forgotten.

Group mix

With the group mix, there really aren't any 'do's and don'ts'. My advice is, if at all possible, get to know the members separately, before introducing them to the group. This way you should be able to tell whether the individuals are likely to get on and work well with one another. I have run groups with only women or men and they have been just as successful as mixed groups; equally, I have run groups where all of the members have been at similar stages in their lives and similar ages, and whilst this had a special benefit, groups where there was diversity in age and background were similarly valuable for different reasons. Having members with a range of disabilities can be helpful during the sessions that spend time discovering how these disabilities have affected them. It can become more challenging for the facilitators if a number of the members have moderate to severe cognitive difficulties; equally, however, it can also be demanding when the group members can only identify with their physical disabilities. Again, knowing your members and how they are likely to react to the other members of the group is paramount to a successful group.

Exclusion criteria

Although the group can benefit all individuals with brain injury, those with particularly poor attention spans, concentration and marked memory difficulties may struggle with the group. Equally, those who have limited or no receptive language skills are not suitable for the group. Expressive language problems may limit an individual's ability to contribute to the group, but this is where having a co-facilitator becomes especially important, as the co-facilitator can help the individuals with expressive language difficulties get their point across, using written language, picture books or 'yes/no' responses. It is necessary for the individual to be aware that they have suffered from a brain injury, otherwise they are unlikely to engage in the group. This group is to increase the awareness of what having a brain injury will mean to their lives, however, if they are not able to understand that they have had a brain injury, they will struggle with the group. Challenging behaviour was not an exclusion criterion, however, in the first session, 'Group Rules' are created and these would be reiterated if a member became aggressive during the group. This is a closed group, so, ideally, all members would be expected to complete all eight sessions. Therefore, individuals who had discharge dates pending within the four weeks of the group would not be included.

Before the first session, there are a few other things that must be considered. First, where will the group take place? As mentioned earlier, I found it most beneficial to run the group in a small room where all the members could sit around one table. This seemed to increase the group's cohesiveness. Second, it helps if there are blank walls in the room so that as the group progresses, the previous week's information can be stuck up as an aide memoire. This way, the Group Rules are accessible to all of the members throughout. This leads nicely to the idea of using a flip-chart. By using a flip-chart and different coloured pens, the group's ideas can be recorded as the members suggest them. It can also be used to help explain some of the more complex ideas, such as what the functions of the different lobes of the brain are. With this in mind, I found it incredibly useful to have a plastic model brain which depicted the different lobes as well as the two hemispheres.

Session 1

What is the Understanding Brain Injury group?

Before this group begins, make sure you are aware of what has happened to each of the group members; this means not only what type of brain injury they have sustained, but also when it occurred, which hospital they were taken to as well as any information on their family, previous jobs and hobbies. This will be needed later in the group to assist the members to fill in the 'My Brain Injury Timeline' section.

At the start of the group, it is useful to have the name of the group and title of the session written on the flip-chart. It helps to ask some basic orientation questions, such as what day, date, month, year and time it is as well as where the group is being held. As the members give the answers to these questions, write them on the flip-chart. This exercise is useful because it helps you ascertain who in the group is most likely to answer an open question such as 'where is this group being held?' Also it will give you an idea about how orientated to time and place the members of the group are.

For this group to work well, all members need to be introduced not only to one another, but also to the idea that they are going to learn about brain injury, their own and other people's, and the effects this can have on their lives in general. This may be the first time many members of the group have met each other, and with this in mind, it is useful to get the members to give their names and tell the group something about themselves. Write the members' names and the facts they give about themselves on a new sheet of the flip-chart so that it can be displayed on the walls for future sessions. Add to this sheet the names of the co-facilitators and include a little something about yourselves as well, in keeping with the group members.

Hand out the worksheets for session 1, explaining that they will receive worksheets each session which will make up the entire workbook. Turning

DOI: 10.4324/9781003441786-3

to the introduction page of the workbook, read aloud the aims of the group. Ask whether there is anything in particular the members would like to discover about their brain injury – write any suggestions on the flip-chart.

Move on to explain how there will be eight sessions; outline briefly what each of these sessions will entail.

Next, it is time for the group to decide on some 'Group Rules'. It is best if the members are asked to come up with rules they would like everyone to follow within the group. However, if they struggle to produce their own list, there are suggestions in the workbook. Write down all of the rules the group agree upon on the flip-chart so that they can be referred to later, if necessary.

After the rules have been agreed upon, go on to discuss the prevalence of brain injury within the UK. I often found this section quite powerful; frequently, the patients were surprised to find out how common brain injury is and how many people are living with the long-term effects of brain injury in the UK alone. On more than one occasion, statements such as 'so we're not alone,' 'I never realised so many people continued life with a brain injury,' 'I thought it was really uncommon … just us … I don't know anyone else with a brain injury' were made after this section of the session. This, I think, starts to help some members feel less isolated and alone.

The next stage is to work on the individuals' timelines. Generally, the members should be given some time to fill in this sheet on their own (or with the help of the facilitators if they cannot read/write). Once everyone has filled in the sheet, the members should be encouraged to share what they have put down with the group. Write this information on the flip-chart.

Time must be spent thinking about what each member sees as their short-, medium- and long-term goals. Again, write these down in the workbook as well as on the flip-chart. Do not worry if the goals appear unrealistic at this stage; allow the individuals to put down what they believe will be achievable within the next month, three months and year.

Finally, recap what has been covered in this session and remind the group of when the next session will be taking place.

Session 1 in summary:

- Items needed for this session include a flip-chart, coloured markers and copies of the worksheets for each participant.

- Get to know your participants before the group starts – what happened to them, when, where they were treated, do they have family, previous jobs, hobbies, etc.
- Write the name of the group and title of the session on the flip-chart
- Ask group orientation questions
- Introduce members to the group, to one another and yourselves
- Hand out worksheets
- Ask whether there is anything in particular the members would like to discover about their brain injuries
- Discuss Group Rules – write these on the flip-chart
- Discuss prevalence of brain injury in the UK
- Work on the group members' timelines
- Discuss each member's timeline and write salient information on the flip-chart
- Go through what each member believes are their short-, medium- and long-term goals– write these down on the worksheets as well as on the flip-chart
- Recap what has been discussed today

Session 2
The brain and brain injury

For this session, the plastic brain mould is really helpful. Also multiple coloured pens can help for illustrating what the different lobes of the brain do.

Start the session with orientation, similar to how you began the first session – ask the members the day, date, month, time and where the group is being held. You should do this at the beginning of every session – although this may seem very basic, it can help to orient your group members to the here and now.

Next, a recap of the first session should be carried out. This will include going through the group rules again as well as reminding the members of their goals. The group rules should be put up on the wall – they should be put up every session.

This session is divided into four separate sections, each one set on a different page of the workbook.

The first section highlights what our brains do; it starts by describing the two hemispheres and explaining what general functions each of the hemispheres are responsible for. This can be found in the workbook. It can be useful to write these on the flip-chart as you describe them. Following this, the areas of the brain are explored. To help with this, the model brain should be handed out and the different lobes pointed out. It can also help to point to where the lobes are on your own head. The workbook contains basic descriptions of the function of each of the lobes, however, when carrying out the group, it can help to go into slightly more detail, although being careful not to swamp the members with information. As you describe what each lobe does, it is really helpful to draw a diagram of the brain, label the lobes and note the most salient parts of what each lobe does. To help, a list has been provided in Appendix 1 of this manual.

DOI: 10.4324/9781003441786-4

The second section of this session focuses on different causes of brain injury. The workbook lists the most common causes of brain injury; however, it may be necessary for you to talk about more obscure forms of brain injury if one of the group members has acquired this. Generally, though, most forms will be covered by the primary five types that are in the workbook – stroke (this includes haemorrhages), hypoxia (heart attack, poisoning, anaphylaxis, electrocution), traumatic (falls, RTAs, assaults), tumours and infections.

The third section involves the members writing about their own brain injury within the workbook. Again, the co-facilitators should enable the members to do this, looking back to session 1 if necessary. Some group members may not know the details of what happened to them or what areas of their brains have been affected. This is where prior knowledge of your group is important. It can also help to talk through what they are finding more difficult since their brain injury – for example, if they have a right-sided hemiparesis, then their brain injury was on the left; if they have memory difficulties, it is likely that they have damaged the temporal lobes. Once all of the members have filled in this sheet, it is advised that they share this with the group and it is written on the flip-chart.

Finally, the group are encouraged to think about what changes they have experienced since their brain injury. These can be broken down into changes that can be seen (physical), changes that cannot be seen (cognitive), changes that other people have noticed and positive things that have helped so far. This can be structured as a table with four columns on the flip-chart for the members to fill in as a group. Once this is done, they can then select the answers they feel most closely reflect their own experiences and enter these in their workbook.

Before the end of the session, recap what has been learnt and state when the next group session will be.

Session 2 in summary

- Items that will be needed for this session include the flip-chart, coloured markers, the worksheets and a model of the brain
- Write the name of the group and title of the session on the flip-chart
- Ask group orientation questions
- Recap the first session

- Describe our brains i.e. the two hemispheres, the different lobes and their functions. Use the plastic model brain to help illustrate the lobes
- Draw a diagram of the brain, label the lobes and note the most salient functions of each
- Discuss the different causes of brain injury and help the group members identify which of these causes applies to them
- Assist the members to write about their own brain injury on the worksheets
- Share this information with the whole group and write it on the flip-chart
- Encourage the group to think about what changes they have experienced since their brain injury (physical, cognitive, aspects others have noticed and positive things that have helped so far). Share these as a group and write it on the flip-chart.
- Recap what has been learnt today.

Session 3
What is rehabilitation?

This session focuses on the different aspects of rehabilitation. If it is possible to have a member of the other rehabilitation therapy teams come in and give a short 10–15 minute discussion about what they do as a Speech and Language Therapist/Occupational Therapist/Physiotherapist that can be very helpful. However, often this will not be possible, either because there are no other therapy teams involved with the clients that are members of the group or because the other teams do not have the resources to spare for this session. When this is the case, the co-facilitators can run this group using the material in the workbook.

At the beginning of the session, orientation should be carried out. After this, the last session should be recapped, answering any questions the members may have regarding the brain and brain injury. The workbook sheets should be handed out.

The first section of this session focuses on explaining what speech and language therapy (SLT) involves. It highlights the fact that Speech and Language therapists try to help people who have suffered brain injury with swallowing and communication. The workbook then breaks this down further into talking, receptive language (listening and reading), expressions and body language, physical changes, thinking changes and swallowing difficulties. The second sheet offers some suggestions of how SLT can help with these difficulties and changes some people with brain injury experience.

Although this can be quite a didactic session, it is possible to make it more interactive by asking the individual members to list any speech or swallowing difficulties they have noticed either in themselves or in other

DOI: 10.4324/9781003441786-5

people they have met who have also suffered a brain injury before going through the list of things SLT can help with. If any of the members have had experience working with SLT, they may be able to suggest some ways that they have been helped before going through this sheet.

The second section deals with explaining what Physiotherapy involves. The workbook lists the different areas physiotherapy affects, including changes in muscle strength, co-ordination, mobility, fatigue, balance, pain and breathing changes. I found it useful to see what the group could produce on their own before relying on what was written in the workbook. To make it more interactive when discussing difficulties with co-ordination, you could see whether the members are able to touch their nose followed by your finger in quick succession or throw bean bags back and forth between the members. Other tasks could involve the members having to grasp an object in a bag and decide what that object is by feel alone (change in fine motor abilities and the sensation of touch) or, with their eyes closed, stretch out their arms in front of them so that they are both level (proprioception – sense of their body in space). These are all tasks that I used in my groups as it broke up the session nicely. To finish this section, ideas on how physiotherapy can help should be discussed.

The third section is about Occupational Therapy (OT). This can often be quite confusing as many people may think this therapy involves re-engaging them in a job. In fact, OT is interested in engaging people in doing the everyday tasks of living – the occupations that we all have to and need to do, whether that is showering, dressing, shopping, cooking, etc., all the way up to having a vocation. Try to have the members list as many occupations as they can think of that an OT may help them achieve and ways that this might be accomplished before looking in the workbook.

The fourth section is neuropsychology. Frequently, many of the members may not have had much input from a neuropsychologist, so they may not know what we do. However, some might have had psychometric assessments conducted at some stage, especially shortly after their brain injury. They may also have seen a psychologist for mood or behavioural issues. If they have not had any experience of what a psychologist can offer, a brief summary is provided in the workbook.

Before the end of the session, recap what has been learnt and state when the next group session will be.

Session 3 in summary

- Items that will be needed for this session include the flip-chart, coloured markers, the worksheets, bean-bags and a bag with small items in it
- Write the name of the group and title of the session on the flip-chart
- Ask group orientation questions
- Recap the second session
- Explain the purpose of Speech and Language Therapy, how it helps with swallowing and communication
- Ask group what difficulties with communicating or swallowing they have noticed within themselves or others
- Go through worksheets on SLT, highlighting some of the suggestions of how SLT can help with these changes after brain injury
- Then, move on to discussing what Physiotherapy involves. Try to get the group to identify as many of these as they can before using the worksheet
- To make the session more interactive, do the activities suggested
- Discuss ideas on how physiotherapy can help an individual after brain injury
- Explain what Occupational Therapy is
- Encourage the members to list as many occupations they can think of that OT may help them achieve and ways that this might be accomplished
- Ask whether anyone in the group has been seen by a psychologist and see whether they can think of reasons why they might be referred to see a psychologist following a brain injury
- Explain what neuropsychologists can do for a person following brain injury
- Recap what has been learnt today

Session 4
Physical changes
after brain injury

The purpose of this session is threefold: first, to increase the group members' understanding of the effects of their brain injury on physical abilities; second, to increase their awareness of the impact of their brain injury on their physical abilities and how this may impact their everyday life, emotions, identity and behaviour; and third, to increase their understanding of the rehabilitation process.

As with the other sessions, start by asking the orientation questions and writing the answers on the flip-chart. Recap what was learnt in the last session, reminding the group what the different therapy teams can offer.

On the flip-chart write 'Physical Changes' in the centre. Ask the members of the group what physical changes they have noticed within themselves as well as within other people who have experienced brain injury. Note these on the flip-chart in a spider diagram format. If the members struggle to produce a list of physical changes on their own, ask questions relating to what they used to do but can no longer do because of the physical difficulties to help highlight these changes (i.e. who used to enjoy riding a bike? Would you be able to do that now? Why not? because of weakness/balance difficulties etc.). Once the group have exhausted their list, check in the workbook and see if there are any further difficulties listed that the group identify with (see Appendix 2 for a more expansive list of physical changes).

Next, ask the group members what these changes make them feel about themselves. Write these responses in a different colour radiating out from the changes. Again, prompt questions might be necessary to get the members really thinking about how they feel when they cannot do something they used to do with ease. Examples of these could be: When you realise you can no longer do X because of your disability, how does that make

DOI: 10.4324/9781003441786-6

you feel? What does it make you think of yourself? These emotions do not have to directly correlate to any one difficulty, rather, they are emotions that may or may not be elicited by any of the difficulties mentioned. Again, once the group think they have mentioned all of the emotions that these changes have elicited, check in the workbook to see if anything has been forgotten.

Following this, the next area of discussion should be on what has helped them cope with these difficulties since their brain injury. These should be written on the spider diagram, radiating out from the emotions, in a different colour pen. These can often be quite difficult to elucidate from the group, as often they may not feel they are coping. Questions that may help in this situation are: what do you do to distract yourself from these thoughts and feelings? How do you deal with these difficulties on a daily basis? As with the list of emotions, each coping strategy does not have to correspond directly to one emotion, rather, this is just a visual representation depicting the many different coping strategies that can help with the emotions and difficulties that occur after brain injury. Once more, when the group think they have given a full account of all strategies they use to help them cope with both the difficulties and the feelings the physical changes have caused, check in the workbook, as there is a page dedicated to this.

Finally, at the bottom of the flip-chart, list suggestions of who the members can turn to for help and advice in yet another colour.

I found it useful to create a computerised copy of the spider diagram that the group constructed so that the members could put it in with the worksheets for this session. Generally, this was done between the sessions and given out at the start of the following session.

See Appendix 3 for an example of the Physical Changes spider diagram.

Session 4 in summary

- Items that will be needed for this session include the flip-chart, coloured markers and the worksheets
- Write the name of the group and title of the session on the flip-chart
- Ask group orientation questions
- Recap the third session
- On the flip-chart, write 'Physical Changes' in the centre

- Ask the members of the group what physical changes they have noticed within themselves as well as in other people who have experienced brain injury
- Note these responses on the flip-chart, radiating out from the central 'Physical Changes' title
- Check the worksheets to see whether there are any further changes the group have not generated but would identify with. Add these to the flip-chart
- Ask the group what these changes make them feel about themselves. Write their responses in a different colour, radiating out from the changes
- Once the group think they have mentioned all of the emotions that these changes elicit, check the worksheet to see if anything has been forgotten
- Ask the group for suggestions of things that have helped them with these difficulties and the way they feel about themselves. Write these coping strategies down, radiating out from the emotions in a different colour pen
- Once the group thinks they have mentioned all the strategies they use to help them cope with both the difficulties and the feelings the physical changes have caused, check the worksheets
- Suggestions of who the members can turn to for help and advice should be written down in yet another colour at the bottom of the flip-chart

Session 5
Thinking changes after brain injury

As with session 4, there are three main objectives to this session: to increase the members' understanding of the effects of their brain injury on their thinking skills, to increase the understanding of the impact of cognitive changes on their everyday life and, once again, to increase their understanding of the rehabilitation process.

As usual, start the session with the orientation questions to regroup the members to the here and now. Go back to the spider diagram that was created in the last session and refresh the group's memory of what was discussed. It can be useful to display this spider diagram on the wall so that the members can refer to it throughout the rest of the sessions.

This time, write 'Thinking Changes' in the centre of the flip-chart. As with the session on physical changes, try to get the group members to generate as many thinking changes as they can independently and write them down emanating from 'Thinking Changes.' Unlike with physical changes, these can be more difficult for the group to produce, as these changes are not always as obvious. It can help to ask them what changes they have noticed in other people, including other members of the group. If this is still a difficulty, it may help to describe some scenarios in which they may struggle due to cognitive deficits and ask whether they have experienced having any problems carrying out these tasks now. Examples of this could include: going grocery shopping and leaving your list at home, listening to an hour-long talk or needing to plan a holiday. Another way of generating ideas could be to ask whether anyone in the group ever finds it hard to do any of the thinking skills we know are likely to have been compromised (see Appendix 4 for a comprehensive list). Once the group have exhausted their list, check in the workbook and see if there are any further difficulties listed that the group identify with.

DOI: 10.4324/9781003441786-7

Following this, ask the group what they believe these changes say about them; how do they feel about the changes; what emotions do these changes elicit? Write these on the flip-chart in a separate colour, spreading out from the list of changes. As with the feelings about physical changes, it is likely that prompt questions will be needed to encourage the group members to think about how they are feeling about their cognitive difficulties. Some people may find this too difficult or painful to do, however, they may be able to think about how other people would feel if they had these problems. Similar to the physical changes, these emotions do not have to directly correlate to any one difficulty, rather, they are emotions that may or may not be elicited by any of the difficulties mentioned. Once the group think they have mentioned all of the ways having these difficulties make them feel, check the workbook to see whether there are any further emotions that the group recognise.

Next, ask the group to generate a list of things that help them cope with both the cognitive deficits as well as the feelings they have in relation to these difficulties. Write these on the flip-chart, in a different colour, radiating out from the feelings about thinking changes as a visual representation of strategies that can assist with the difficulties and the emotions these changes cause. These can range from memory aids, notebooks for planning, taking regular breaks when working, to talking to others or doing something enjoyable. At this point, the same type of questions can be asked as in session 4. When the group think they have given a full account of all strategies they use to help them cope with both the difficulties and the feelings the thinking changes have caused, check in the workbook, as there is a page dedicated to this.

Finally, at the bottom of the flip-chart, suggestions of people who the members can turn to for help and advice should be written down in yet another colour.

See Appendix 5 for an example of the Thinking Changes spider diagram.

Session 5 in summary

- Items that will be needed for this session include the flip-chart, coloured markers and the worksheets
- Write the name of the group and title of the session on the flip-chart
- Ask group orientation questions

- Recap the fourth session
- On the flip-chart, write 'Thinking Changes' in the centre
- Try to get the group to generate as many thinking changes as possible that they have either noticed within themselves or in other people who have suffered from brain injury
- Note these on the flip-chart, radiating out from the central 'Thinking changes' title
- Check the worksheets to see whether there are any further changes the group have not generated but would identify with. Add these to the flip-chart
- Ask the group what these changes make them feel about themselves. Write their responses in a different colour, radiating out from the changes
- Once the group think they have mentioned all of the emotions that these changes elicit from them, check the worksheet to see if anything has been forgotten
- Ask the group for suggestions of things that have helped them with these difficulties and the way they feel about themselves. Write these coping strategies radiating out from the emotions in a different colour pen
- Once the group thinks they have mentioned all the strategies they use to help them cope with both the difficulties and the feelings the thinking changes have caused, check with the worksheets
- Suggestions of who the members can turn to for help and advice should be written down in yet another colour at the bottom of the flip-chart
- Recap what has been learnt in the session

Session 6
Mood and behaviour changes after brain injury

As with the previous two sessions, the main objective to this session is to increase the individuals' acknowledgement and understanding of the impact of their brain injury, this time on their mood and behaviour, and how this in turn effects their everyday life.

As with the previous sessions, start the group with the orientation questions, followed by a short summary of session 5 using the spider diagram that was created to remind the members of what was discussed. Again, stick this diagram on the wall alongside the diagram from session 4.

Once the members have been reminded of what they have learnt so far, write on the flip-chart 'Mood and Behaviour Changes.' Ask the members what changes in mood or behaviour they have noticed within themselves or in other people with brain injury. Write these changes on the flip-chart. As with thinking changes, these can be more difficult – it may help if the facilitators suggest some situations in which the members find their behaviours or mood have changed, for example, when around strangers, when attempting to do something new or when surrounded by family. Once they think they have mentioned all of the mood and behaviour changes they have noticed within themselves and others, check through the workbook, which highlights the most common changes.

Next, as with the past sessions, enquire how these changes make the members feel about themselves; what do the changes say about them. Write these down on the flip-chart, radiating from the list of changes (each emotion does not need to correlate to a change directly). Again, just as with the feelings about physical and thinking changes, prompt questions may be needed to encourage the group members to think about how they feel regarding any alterations they are experiencing to their mood and behaviours. Examples of

DOI: 10.4324/9781003441786-8

these could include: 'when you realise you are experiencing this behaviour, how does it make you feel? When you notice your mood, what emotions are you feeling'? Use the workbook to see whether there are any emotions or feelings that the group identify with which they have not already produced.

Ask the group what they do to help them cope with the changes in their mood and behaviours as well as the feelings that these changes elicit. Write these on the flip-chart, in a different colour, spreading out from the feelings about the changes, again as a visual representation, as opposed to each coping strategy needing to line up with an emotion or specific difficulty. Questions that may help generate coping strategies the members use include 'what helps distract you from these feelings? What do you do to reduce these emotions? What do you do to stop your behaviour?' Once the members feel they have exhausted their own list of coping strategies, look in the workbook and see if there are any further strategies that the group identify with that can be added to the spider diagram.

As with the other sessions, a list of people who the members can turn to for support with their mood and behavioural changes should be written down in a different colour.

See Appendix 6 for an example of the Mood and Behaviour changes spider diagram.

Session 6 in summary

- Items that will be needed for this session include the flip-chart, coloured markers and the worksheets
- Write the name of the group and title of the session on the flip-chart
- Ask group orientation questions
- Recap the fifth session
- On the flip-chart write 'Mood and Behaviour Changes' in the centre
- Try to get the group to generate as many mood or behaviour changes as possible that they have either noticed within themselves or in other people who have suffered from brain injury
- Note these down on the flip-chart, radiating out from the central 'Mood and Behaviour Changes' title
- Check the worksheets to see whether there are any further changes the group have not generated but would identify with. Add these to the flip-chart

- Ask the group what these changes make them feel about themselves. Write their responses in a different colour, radiating out from the changes
- Once the group think they have mentioned all of the emotions that these changes elicit from them, check the worksheet to see if anything has been forgotten
- Ask the group for suggestions of things that have helped them with these difficulties and the way they feel about themselves. Write down these coping strategies radiating out from the emotions in a different colour pen
- Once the group thinks they have mentioned all the strategies they use to help them cope with both the difficulties and the feelings the mood and behaviour changes have caused, check with the worksheets
- Suggestions of who the members can turn to for help and advice should be written down in yet another colour at the bottom of the flip-chart
- Recap what has been learnt in the session

Session 7
Lifestyle changes after brain injury

This is the last session which will be based around using the spider diagram format. As with the previous three sessions, its emphasis is on trying to encourage the members to identify the changes to their lifestyle the brain injury will have caused. The aim for this session is to help the members understand how their brain injury has affected their lifestyle, aiding them in recognising the feelings they have about these changes and finally facilitating their discovery of coping strategies for both the changes as well as the emotions they feel regarding these differences.

Start the group with the usual orientation, which should be written on a sheet of the flip-chart. Go back over the last session to remind the members of what was discussed; do this by using the spider diagram which was created during the last session. Pin this up on the wall.

On a new sheet of the flip-chart write 'Lifestyle Changes.' Ask the group what changes they have experienced in their lifestyle since their brain injury. If this group is being run in an inpatient setting, it may be necessary to ask them what they think will have changed once they have been discharged. If the members struggle to think of any areas of their lives that will have changed, ask prompt questions such as: 'how do you think you will manage work?' and 'What changes do you imagine there might be within your role at home?' Write all of the changes that the group produce on the flip-chart, radiating from Lifestyle Changes. A list of lifestyle changes has been incorporated in Appendix 7 to help.

From here, as with the previous sessions, feelings about these lifestyle changes need to be addressed. Enquire what emotions the members feel when thinking about the lifestyle changes they have had to deal with or are expecting to need to deal with. Write this list of feelings on the spider

DOI: 10.4324/9781003441786-9

diagram, spreading out from the changes. As with the other diagrams, the emotions do not need to directly correlate to a specific change.

Next, ask the group what coping strategies they use to help with the changes to their lifestyle as well as with the feelings that these changes cause. Often, the individuals may not have had to deal with the actual changes yet (i.e. they are still in hospital but envision not being able to drive anymore as being problematic and frustrating), thus, conceiving coping strategies may be difficult but will be ultimately useful in the long term. Again, the same type of questions as in the other sessions can be of use here. This section is particularly important as it looks at how the members are going to cope with their lifestyle changes in the future. Write down all suggestions on the flip-chart, emanating from the emotions, as with all of the other spider diagrams.

As with the other sessions, a list of people who the members can turn to for advice and support with their lifestyle changes should be written down in a different colour.

See Appendix 8 for an example of the Lifestyle Changes spider diagram.

Session 7 in summary

- Items that will be needed for this session include the flip-chart, coloured markers and the worksheets
- Write the name of the group and title of the session on the flip-chart
- Ask group orientation questions
- Recap the sixth session
- On the flip-chart, write 'Lifestyle Changes' in the centre
- Try to get the group to generate as many lifestyle changes as possible that they have either noticed within themselves or in other people who have suffered from brain injury
- Note these down on the flip-chart, radiating out from the central 'Lifestyle Changes' title
- Check the worksheets to see whether there are any further changes the group have not generated but would identify with. Add these to the flip-chart
- Ask the group what these changes make them feel about themselves. Write their responses in a different colour, radiating out from the changes
- Once the group think they have mentioned all of the emotions that these changes elicit from them, check the worksheet to see if anything has been forgotten

- Ask the group for suggestions of things that have helped them with these difficulties and the way they feel about themselves. Write these coping strategies down, radiating out from the emotions in a different colour pen
- Once the group thinks they have mentioned all the strategies they use to help them cope with both the difficulties and the feelings the lifestyle changes have caused, check with the worksheets
- Suggestions of who the members can turn to for help and advice should be written down in yet another colour at the bottom of the flip-chart
- Recap what has been learnt in the session

Session 8
My goals for the future

This is the final session of the group, therefore it will mainly summarise the previous weeks, recapping what the members have learnt over the past seven sessions. It will also dedicate some time to looking at what the members chose as their short-, medium- and long-term goals in the initial session and see whether the individuals still see those goals as being realistic in the period of time they set for themselves.

Once orientation has been completed, take all four spider diagrams and display them on the walls so that they can be seen easily by all members of the group. Ask whether the members can see any resemblances between the four diagrams – do they see any similarities in the way that their difficulties make them feel? How about similarities in the way that they cope with these changes and emotions? Next, see whether the members can identify any similarities in whom they can turn to for assistance, both within a rehabilitation setting and within the community (family, friends, faith, etc.).

Ask each member what their goals were at the beginning of the UBI group; write these on the flip-chart. Turn to the booklet; in session 8, there is a page entitled 'Reviewing My Goals.' Ask the group members to fill in what they had chosen to be their short-, medium- and long-term goals during session 1, in the relevant spaces. Discuss with each of the members how they feel they are managing these goals; ask whether they think they overestimated or underestimated their abilities and how long the rehabilitation process would take. Ask them to write what progress they have made so far towards each goal in the relevant space.

Next, discuss with the group what goals are still important to them. Sometimes what seemed very important at the beginning of the group sessions will no longer seem so, because of this, it is essential that each group

DOI: 10.4324/9781003441786-10

member think about what goals they still feel are important, and more crucially, achievable. On the sheet entitled 'Moving Towards My Future Goals' the members should write down what their goals for the future are, along with what steps they will need to take to achieve these goals.

Finally, all of the previous group sessions should be summarised; this is where the flip-chart sheets come in handy for reminding the group about what was discussed in sessions 1–7 – the visual representation of this material works as a memory aid.

At the very end of the final session, hand out the certificate for attending the Understanding Brain Injury Group (see Appendix 9).

Session 8 in summary

- Items that will be needed for this session include the flip-chart, coloured markers, the worksheets and the group certificates
- Write the name of the group and title of the session on the flip-chart
- Ask group orientation questions
- Recap the seventh session
- Stick all four spider diagrams on the walls so that they can be seen easily by all members of the group
- Ask whether there are any resemblances between the four diagrams – do they see any similarities in the way their difficulties make them feel? Similarities in the way they cope with these feelings and difficulties?
- Return to the goals made at the beginning of the UBI group. Write these on the flip-chart.
- Ask the group members to fill in their short-, medium- and long-term goals on the worksheet on the page entitled 'Reviewing My Goals'
- Discuss with each of the members how they feel they are managing these goals; ask whether they think they overestimated or underestimated their abilities and how long the rehabilitation process would take
- Ask the members to write what progress they have made so far towards each goal in the relevant space
- Discuss which goals are still important to the group. On the sheet entitled 'Moving Towards My Future Goals,' the members should write down their goals for the future along with what steps they will need to achieve these goals
- Summarise all of the previous UBI sessions
- Hand out the Certificate of Attendance

29

Areas of the brain

Right hemisphere: Controls left side of the body

Creative aspects – responsible for rhythm, spatial awareness, colour, imagination, daydreaming, holistic awareness and dimension.

Left hemisphere: Controls right side of the body

Logical brain – responsible for words, logic, numbers, analysis, lists, linearity and sequencing.

Frontal lobe: Positioned at the foremost region of the cerebral cortex.

Involved in: motor functions, decision-making, planning, problem solving, reasoning, judgement, impulse control, personality, attention, organisational abilities, motivation and regulation of emotions.

Parietal lobe: Positioned towards the top and back of the cerebral cortex.

Involved in: integrating sensory information from various parts of the body, knowledge of numbers and their relations, manipulation of objects, processing information related to touch, visuospatial processing.

Temporal lobe: Positioned to the side of the cerebral cortex.

Involved in: auditory perception, memory, speech, comprehension, emotional responses, visual perception.

Occipital lobe: Positioned at the back of the cerebral cortex.

Involved in visual processing.

Appendix

2

List of physical changes

Difficulties with:

- Sitting
- Balance
- Standing
- Walking
- Weakness
- Movement
- Tiredness
- Fatigue
- Pain
- Using arm/hand
- Vision
- Hearing
- Muscle tension
- Muscle tone
- Co-ordination
- Swallowing
- Dizziness
- Speech
- Appetite change
- Loss of sensation
- Incontinence
- Epilepsy

Appendix 3

Example spider diagram of physical changes

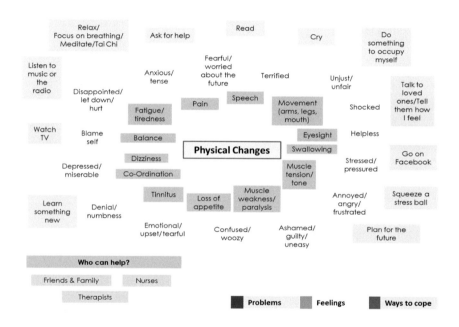

Relax/Focus on breathing/Meditate/Tai Chi

Ask for help

Read

Cry

Do something to occupy myself

Listen to music or the radio

Anxious/tense

Fearful/worried about the future

Terrified

Unjust/unfair

Talk to loved ones/Tell them how I feel

Disappointed/let down/hurt

Fatigue/tiredness

Pain

Speech

Movement (arms, legs, mouth)

Shocked

Watch TV

Blame self

Balance

Physical Changes

Eyesight

Helpless

Dizziness

Swallowing

Go on Facebook

Depressed/miserable

Co-Ordination

Muscle tension/tone

Stressed/pressured

Tinnitus

Loss of appetite

Muscle weakness/paralysis

Annoyed/angry/frustrated

Squeeze a stress ball

Learn something new

Denial/numbness

Emotional/upset/tearful

Confused/woozy

Ashamed/guilty/uneasy

Plan for the future

Who can help?

Friends & Family

Nurses

Therapists

◼ Problems   ◼ Feelings   ◼ Ways to cope

Appendix

4

List of cognitive changes

Difficulties with:

- Memory – short- and long-term
- Retrograde amnesia
- Anterograde amnesia
- Planning
- Problem solving
- Decision making
- Organising
- Reasoning
- Attention
- Concentration
- Speed of information processing
- Visuospatial abilities
- Perceptual abilities
- Speaking
- Comprehension
- Reading
- Writing
- Confusion
- Disorientation
- Understanding
- Impulsivity
- Impatience

Example spider diagram of thinking ability changes

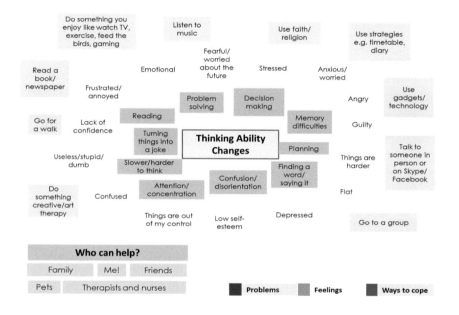

Example spider diagram of mood and behaviour changes

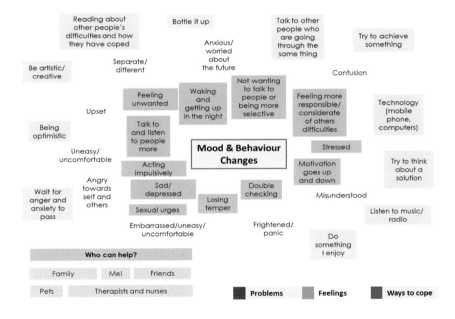

Reading about other people's difficulties and how they have coped

Bottle it up

Talk to other people who are going through the same thing

Try to achieve something

Be artistic/creative

Separate/different

Anxious/worried about the future

Confusion

Feeling unwanted

Waking and getting up in the night

Not wanting to talk to people or being more selective

Feeling more responsible/considerate of others difficulties

Technology (mobile phone, computers)

Upset

Talk to and listen to people more

Mood & Behaviour Changes

Stressed

Being optimistic

Uneasy/uncomfortable

Acting impulsively

Motivation goes up and down

Try to think about a solution

Angry towards self and others

Sad/depressed

Double checking

Misunderstood

Wait for anger and anxiety to pass

Losing temper

Sexual urges

Listen to music/radio

Embarrassed/uneasy/uncomfortable

Frightened/panic

Do something I enjoy

Who can help?		
Family	Me!	Friends
Pets	Therapists and nurses	

Problems   Feelings   Ways to cope

Appendix

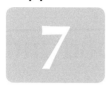

List of lifestyle changes

Difficulties with:

- Daily activities
  - Showering
  - Dressing
  - Toileting
- Cooking
- Shopping
- Housing
- Driving
- Travelling
- Family roles
- Relationships
- Friendships

Example spider diagram of lifestyle changes

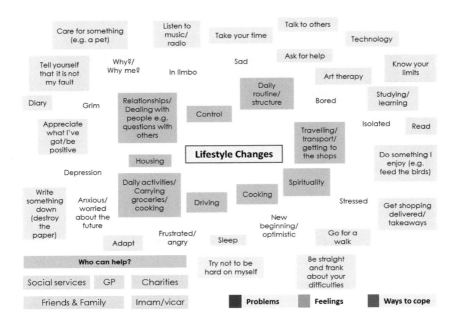

Appendix

9

Certificate
of attendance

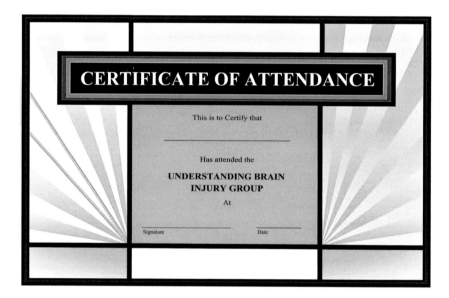

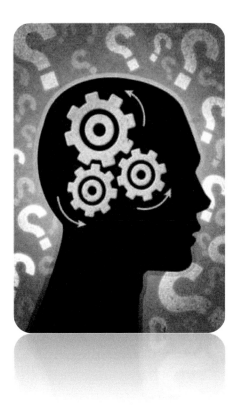

**Understanding
Brain Injury
Group**

Date:

Name:

Introduction

This group is about:

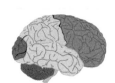

- Learning more about the brain

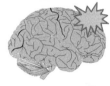

- Understanding what brain injury is

- Learning about the effects of brain injury

- Thinking about what you can do to cope with these changes

Contents

There are 8 group sessions:

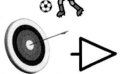

Session 1:
Introduction to UBI Group

In this session we will:

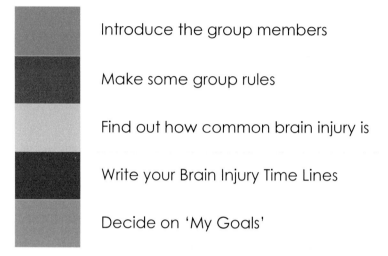

Introduce the group members

Make some group rules

Find out how common brain injury is

Write your Brain Injury Time Lines

Decide on 'My Goals'

Group Rules

Here are some suggested group rules:

- Be on time
- Let everyone have the same time to speak
- Don't speak over other people
- Don't swear or make inappropriate comments
- Listen and respect each other
- Be aware of privacy. Please do not speak about the group outside of the sessions.
- Please do not use your mobile phone.
- Do you have any other rules to add?

_____

_____

_____

_____

How Common is Brain Injury?

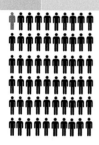

Out of all the people in the UK:

- About **1 in 60** people in the UK go to A&E because of head injuries every year

Out of these 1 million people:

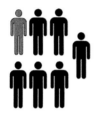

- About **1 in 7** of these people stay in hospital because their injuries are more serious

Across the UK:

- About half a million people (500,000) are living with long term problems because of brain injury

Types of Brain Injuries:

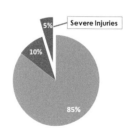

- Minor or Mild: about 85% of all brain injuries

- Moderate: about 10% of all brain injuries

- Severe: about 5% of all brain injuries

More men than women have brain injuries.

44

My Brain Injury Timeline

<u>My Life Before My Brain Injury:</u>

My job & hobbies:

_____

_____

My family:

_____

_____

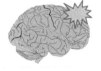

<u>My Brain Injury:</u>

What happened?

_____

_____

When did this happen?

_____

_____

What happened next?

_____

_____

<u>What changes have I noticed since my head injury?</u>

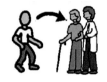 Physical changes:

_____

_____

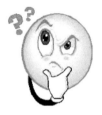 Thinking Changes:

_____

_____

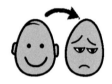 Mood & Behaviour Changes:

_____

_____

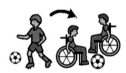 Lifestyle Changes:

_____

_____

Key Point: Rehabilitation is to help you cope with these changes.

Different therapists will work with you to help you overcome any difficulties you now have

My Goals

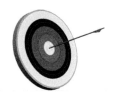

<u>What I need to do to help my recovery:</u>

Short Term Goals (in the next month?)

_____

_____

Medium Term Goals (in the next three months?)

_____

_____

Long Term Goals (in the next year?)

_____

_____

_____

Session 2:

The Brain and Brain Injuries

In this session we'll look at:

  The Two Halves of the Brain

  The Areas of the Brain

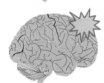 Different types of Brain Injury

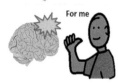 My Brain Injury

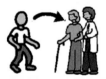 Changes since my Brain Injury

The Two Halves of the Brain

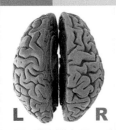

The Brain has two halves or "hemispheres"

These are called the:

- **Left** Hemisphere
- **Right** Hemisphere

Movement

These control the movements of the opposite side of the body:

- The **Left** Hemisphere controls your **Right** side
- The **Right** Hemisphere controls your **Left** side

Thinking Abilities

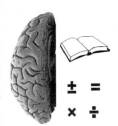

The **Left** Hemisphere is involved with:

- Language (example: Speaking, Reading)
- Logical Thinking (example: Maths, Rules)

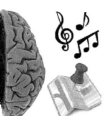

The **Right** Hemisphere is involved with:

- Visual abilities (example: Drawing, Maps)
- Music (example: Singing, Speech Intonation)

The Areas of the Brain

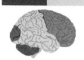

The Brain is divided into four main areas.
These are called the "Lobes"

The **Occipital** Lobe
- Vision / Sight

The **Parietal** Lobe
- Touch / Sensations
- Perception & making sense of the world

The **Temporal** Lobe
- Memory
- Language

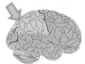

The **Frontal** Lobe
- Executive Abilities (Organisation, Planning)
- Mood and Behaviour ('Personality')

There are two other areas which are at the base of the brain.

The **Cerebellum**
- Balance
- Co-ordination of movement

The **Brain Stem**
- Vital Functions (heartbeat, breathing, blood pressure)

Different Types of Brain Injury

Key Fact: The brain needs oxygen to work properly. Oxygen is like the 'fuel of the brain'. Blood carries oxygen around the body and brain in blood vessels. Brain injury is caused when parts of the brain do not get enough blood.

Stroke

A stroke is when blood does not get to a particular part of the brain.

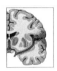

A stroke can happen when:

- A blood vessel gets blocked
- A blood vessel bursts and the blood leaks out

Hypoxia

When not enough oxygen gets to the brain it is called hypoxia. Really severe hypoxia is called anoxia.

This is often caused by heart attacks, but there are many other causes including poisoning, near drowning and suicide attempts.

Traumatic Brain Injury

The brain can be injured by a blow to the head:

Closed head injury: this is a blow to the outside of the head, such as in a car accident or fall

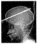

Open head injury: this is when the injury gets into the brain itself, for example due to a gunshot or piercing injury

Tumours

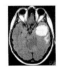

Tumours are when cells grow abnormally. This leads to a mass of extra tissue inside the brain.

Tumours take up extra space inside the skull and can put pressure on the brain. They are sometimes cancerous.

Infections

The brain can become infected; this is called encephalitis

My Brain Injury

What happened?

_____

When did it happen?

_____

Where is my brain injury?

This might be one place or many places

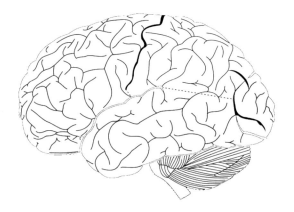

What hemisphere was most affected?

Left hemisphere   **Right** hemisphere

Which lobes of the brain were most affected?

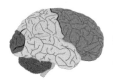

Occipital Lobe   **Parietal** Lobe

Temporal Lobe   **Frontal** Lobe

Changes since my Brain Injury

<u>Since my brain injury happened:</u>

Are there any changes that I can see?

_____

_____

_____

Are there any changes I cannot see (such as my thinking abilities)?

_____

_____

_____

What changes have other people noticed?

_____

_____

_____

What positive things have helped?

_____

_____

_____

Session 3:
What is Rehabilitation?

This session includes:

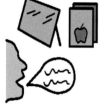

Speech and Language Therapy: what difficulties can they help with and how do they help?

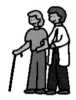

Physiotherapy: what difficulties can they help with and how do they help?

Occupational Therapy: what difficulties can they help with and how do they help?

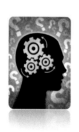

Neuropsychology: what difficulties can they help with and how do they help?

54

Difficulties Speech and Language Therapy (SLT) help with:

SLT is about helping people communicate and swallow

Talking

- You may have weak lips or a weak tongue
- You may find it difficult to think/find the right words

Information going in:

- You may find it hard to understand what other people are saying.
- You may find it difficult to pay attention to large amounts of information.

Writing

- It can be hard to hold a pen
- It can be difficult to find the word you want to write
- You may find it difficult to spell words

Expressions and Body Language

- You may have difficulty accurately understanding other people's emotions.

Physical Changes

- You may have hearing problems
- You may find it hard to move your body or face

Thinking Changes

- You may find it difficult to remember conversations
- You may find it hard to pay attention and concentrate.

Swallowing Changes

- You may find it hard to swallow and be on a special diet

Feelings about communication problems

It is common for people to feel upset about problems they have with communication. These include:

- Frustration, embarrassment, tiredness or sadness

How can SLT help?

Here are some things that can help:

- **Listen carefully** when someone is talking to you. **Look at their faces**. Ask people to repeat and/or slow down.

- **Move to a quiet place** to talk or listen. Turn the TV or radio down.

- **Write down** information you need to remember.

- **Think** about what you want to say **before** saying it.

- Use **short** sentences.

Go! VS
Please start now.

- **Use your hands and facial expressions** when talking.

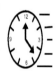

- Take your time. **Don't rush!**

- **Practice the strategies** that your SLT teaches you to use

Difficulties Physiotherapy can help with:

Physiotherapy helps patients build up physical abilities:

Change in Muscle Strength

- One side of the body may become weaker than the other
- This can make daily tasks difficult. For example: holding a cup or brushing your teeth.

Change in co-ordination

- Poor co-ordination means that it is difficult to make successful and smooth movements

Tense Muscles

- Brain Injury can cause increased muscle tone (very tense muscles)
- Muscles can be painful and difficult to stretch

Mobility

- People may find it hard to move independently, especially staying safe and not falling

Some examples are:

- Changing positions in bed.
- Moving from one chair to another.
- Using a wheelchair
- Learning how to walk again

Fatigue and Tiredness

- Brain Injury can cause muscle weakness, this means that we are more likely to become tired

Balance

Reasons why balance may be affected after brain injury include:

- Problems with your inner ear - this is important for balance.

- Sensory problems are important, such as vision and having a sense of your body in space
- Changes in thinking ability can also affect balance

Permanent body changes

- Sometimes, muscles and tendons in the body can shorten after brain injury. These are called *contractures*.
- **Pain**: Some people feel pain more easily or it may seem more intense.
- **Numbness**: Other people may not feel very much at all, even when holding an object.
- **Temperature**: Brain injury can change how we feel heat and cold.
- **Pressure**: Some people find it difficult to tell how hard something is touching then.

Breathing changes

- Shortness of Breath
- Coughing
- Wheezing
- Chest infections

How can Physiotherapy help?

- Physiotherapy can help you by providing you with a series of exercises to improve your strength, endurance, mobility, flexibility, posture and balance.

- If you aren't able to move your muscles yourself they can actively move them for you.

- They can use electrical stimulation to help you regain the use of your muscles

- They may provide supports to aid you with your mobility, posture and balance.

Difficulties Occupational Therapy can help with

Occupational therapy is about helping people to do the everyday things they want and need to do.

It supports people to take part in everyday living. There are two main ways in which occupational therapy helps people with everyday tasks:
- Supports people to improve their abilities
- Changes the environment to make it easier to do everyday tasks

Occupational Therapists (OTs) help people with all types of illness, injury or disability. They support people to become as independent as possible in everyday life.

OTs focus on activities and tasks which a person finds useful and meaningful.

OTs help with many everyday activities. For example:

- Washing and dressing
- Eating and drinking
- Shopping
- Cooking
- Adapting houses
- Going back to work

How does OT help?

Re-learning how you used to do things

Your OT will help you practice day to day activities. Doing these will gradually build up your skills and confidence over time.

Learning new ways of doing things

Another way OTs help is to support you to do things in a different way, to make them easier.

- Writing shopping lists before going shopping
- Using calendars or diaries to plan your days
- Using your stronger hand for everyday tasks

Special Equipment and gadgets

If it is difficult to learn a new way of doing a task, sometimes it is useful to use special equipment

- Using a grab rail, if climbing stairs is difficult
- Cutlery with a large handle if gripping is hard

Difficulties Neuropsychology can help with

Cognition or thinking abilities

- Orientation.
- Attention and concentration.
- Memory.
- Perception.
- Language.
- Planning.
- Impulsivity.

Mood

- Sadness.
- Depression.
- Anxiety.
- Anger.

Challenging Behaviour
- Agitation.
- Verbal aggression.
- Physical aggression.
- Threatening behaviour.
- Sexual inappropriateness

Specific Issues with Recovery
- Adjustment.
- Coping with Loss.
- Change in your Role.

We also work with family members and other outside agencies preparing for when you leave here.

How can Neuropsychology help?

Neuropsychology can help by completing assessments with you, which will help us understand your strengths and what areas of thinking you might be having some difficulty with.

Once we know where your strengths lie we can use these to compensate for the areas you are having more difficulty in; for example if you are having difficulty remembering routines, but are able to read and write, then we may help you create a notebook or calendar to detail your routines.

We can also help you with any emotional concerns you may be having, whether that be feeling low, anxious, worried about the future or feeling angry.

We can work with people close to you such as your family to help them understand more about your brain injury and we can support them and you if you are having any difficulties.

We work alongside other members of the team to try and understand why someone might be challenging after a brain injury e.g. hitting other people or shouting out. We then help them and the team develop new ways of interacting to manage and/or reduce this behaviour.

Session 4:
Physical Changes after Brain Injury

This session includes:

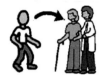 Common Physical Changes

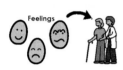 Feelings about Physical Changes

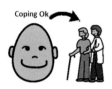 Coping with Physical Changes

Common Physical Difficulties

Brain injuries can lead to physical problems; these depend on where exactly the brain injury is

Tiredness

It is common to feel tired more easily after brain injury.

- Some people find they can't do as much exercise
- Many people need to take more breaks and rests when recovering from a brain injury

Muscle Weakness

After brain injury, it is common to have weakness in our muscles (legs, arms, face)

- This is often on one side of the body more than the other

Co-ordination

It is common for brain injuries to lead to:

- Problems co-ordinating movements, such as making a cup of tea
- Problems controlling movement, such as difficulties writing or staying still

Walking and Movement

Many people are less mobile after brain injuries. For example:

- Some people find it difficult to move at all and need help to roll in bed or sit up
- Some people are able to move, but find it difficult to walk or get up from a chair

Increased Muscle Tone

This is when muscles are tense and difficult to relax

- This can make it difficult to stretch muscles
- It can be painful

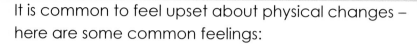

Feelings about Physical Changes

It is common to feel upset about physical changes –
here are some common feelings:

Frustration

When people cannot do as much, they often feel
frustrated. Here are some things that can lead to this:

- Not being able to get out of bed yourself
- Feeling tired after going for a short walk

Anger

Some people can feel angry about their physical
problems.

- They might be angry at the world or angry at God
  because of their brain injury
- Some people become angry with the people
  around them, such as family or carers

Sadness

Realising you cannot do as much as you used to can
lead people to feel sad or low.

- Some people focus on things they can no longer
  do, such as walking or playing sport
- This can make people feel very low and not want
  to do much at all

Deny Problems or Feel Numb

Some people find it very difficult to think about the
problems they have, especially early on

- Some people might try not to think about these, or
  "play them down"
- Other people might feel overwhelmed and aren't
  able to think about their problems

Coping with Physical Changes

Physical problems after brain injury are common and can make people feel upset; however people do cope well with these.

Here are some things people find help them cope.

Do things you enjoy!

It is important to keep doing things that you enjoy and can do. For example:

- Listening to music, watching television or reading
- Spending time with other people, such as friends and family

Find other ways to do it!

If physical problems are holding you back, it can help to find other ways to do what you want.

- You could try taking more breaks and giving yourself more time to do the task

- You can use some equipment to help or support you, for example a walking aid or wheelchair.

Ask Other People for Support!

Sometimes physical problems mean we cannot do something by ourselves, and so we need to ask for help:

Take part in Rehabilitation!

People do recover from some physical difficulties. Physiotherapy and other rehab helps recovery by:

- Exercising to become stronger, for example moving your legs or making your grip stronger
- Learning new ways of doing things and new skills, for example using a 'rota stand'

Session 5:
Thinking Changes after Brain Injury

This session includes:

   Common Thinking Ability Changes

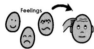   Feelings about Cognitive Changes

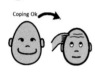   Coping with Cognitive Changes

Common Thinking Difficulties

The brain is responsible for our thinking abilities. These are also called 'cognitive abilities'

Brain injuries can lead to cognitive problems

Again, the exact problems depend on where the brain is damaged, so everyone is different

Slower Thinking Speed

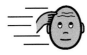

This is called reduced "processing speed" meaning that it takes longer to take in and make sense of information

This is very common after brain injuries

Difficulties this may lead to in daily life include:

- Not being able to keep up with others' conversation
- Taking longer to do something compared to before your brain injury
- Not taking all the information in, so that you never get the chance to learn it

Memory

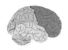

Memory problems are linked with injuries in the **Frontal** and Temporal Lobes.

Memory problems can affect:

- Recently learned information
- Older information
- Remembering to do something in the future

Memories come in two main types:

- Explicit Memories: Information you have conscious access to

- Implicit Memories: Knowledge you do not need to consciously access (example: such as how to brush your teeth)

This means that sometimes, people with brain injuries can carry on doing daily tasks, but they find it difficult to adapt to new situations and learn new information.

"Executive" Abilities

Solving new problems involves a lot of different thinking abilities, most of these are in the **Frontal** Lobes

These are referred to as "Executive Functions" because they are like the executive board of a company that oversee all the other abilities
Some examples of executive abilities include:

- Planning before and during tasks
- Organising things
- Solving problems that come up
- Starting actions at the right time

- Stopping actions when needed
- Dividing your attention between different tasks

A good example is planning a journey by public transport as you use most of these abilities to do this

Language

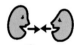

The **Left** Hemisphere is most important for language, but **Right** Hemisphere damage can cause subtle difficulties (example: the 'music' or tone of speech)

These include making ourselves understood (Expressive) and understanding other people (Receptive)
Making ourselves understood includes:

- Speaking (words and grammar)
- Writing
- Non-verbal speech (tone of voice, speed)
- Non-verbal communication (Body Language)

Understanding other people includes:

- Understanding speech

- Reading
- Making sense of what people mean even when they don't say it (social inferencing)

Awareness of Difficulties

The brain is also important for making sense of what has happened to us.

Sometimes, brain injury can cause problems with being aware of our difficulties.

This lack of awareness is normally a mix of:

- Changes in the brain because of brain injury
- Avoiding thoughts about difficulties

This is really important. If people do not understand that they have problems, it can be difficult for them to find solutions for these problems.

People with difficulties with awareness can:

- Say that they don't have any problems at all
- Report some problems, such as physical changes, but not others, such as thinking changes

- Feel like they do not belong in hospital
- Feel like they should not have to work with rehabilitation therapists

Feelings about Cognitive Changes

Cognitive problems have a big impact on our lives; these can be very frustrating as times

It is common to feel upset about these changes; however everyone reacts in their own way.

Here are some common feelings:

Confusion

Difficulties with thinking abilities make the world seem a confusing place. Some examples are:

- Not being aware of exactly where you are, or how you got here, because of memory problems
- Not being able to:
  - understand what other people mean
  - make sense of what is happening

Worry and Anxiety (Nervousness)

Cognitive difficulties can make it difficult to make sense of the world or predict what will happen. This uncertainty and doubt often leads to anxiety. Some examples are:

- Feeling uncertain about what is happening, because it is difficult to remember things
- Worry about how you will manage independently when it is difficult to carry out day-to-day tasks

Frustration & Anger

Cognitive difficulties can be really frustrating, for example:

- Getting frustrated and angry because other people seem to be on a different page to you
- Finding it difficult to communicate things that you need

Sadness

Cognitive problems can lead people to feel low, often because they're aware of the things they can no longer do

Coping with Cognitive Changes

Cognitive problems after brain injury are common and these do not always go away; but people can and do cope with these:

Use Strategies

There are many skills you can learn to help overcome cognitive difficulties:

- Memory Problems: try memory strategies, i.e. anagrams, making stories out of information or picturing it
- Poor Organisation: learn skills to break tasks down into small steps, with checklists to keep on track

Use Supports and Gadgets

Many people have some memory and organisation difficulties. This means that everyone can benefit from helpful strategies.

There are many pieces of equipment available that you can use to help with cognitive difficulties.

iPad

- Simple aids: Notebooks and calendars
- Gadgets: Electronic organisers (mobile phones, iPads) and alarms

Ask other people for support

Sometimes it can be difficult to manage new tasks on your own:

- Ask your Psychologist or Occupational Therapist for help with memory or organisation
- Ask your Speech and Language Therapist for help with language and communication problems
- Ask your family or friends for help

Session 6:
Mood & Behaviour Changes after Brain Injury

This session includes:

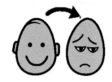 Common Mood Changes

  Feelings about Mood Changes

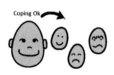 Coping with Mood Changes

Common Mood & Behavioural Difficulties

 The brain controls our mood and behaviour; injury can lead to difficulties depending on where the brain is injured

Rapid Changes in mood

Some people find that their mood changes more rapidly:

- They become angry very quickly and find it difficult to control or manage their temper

- They may find that their mood changes rapidly, crying or laughing all of a sudden.

Sadness

Many people find themselves feeling low or depressed; this can be quite normal but can also lead to feelings of demotivation and apathy.

Anxiety

There may be an increase in worries after a brain injury and these can interfere in your rehabilitation

Acting Impulsively

Many people behave or think impulsively after brain injury.

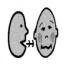
- Inappropriate behaviour: Acting without thinking can make other people uncomfortable or embarrassed. For example, making a sexual comment to someone.

- Rude language: When people are impulsive they can be rude or abusive.

Repeated Behaviour

 After brain injury, people can get stuck on some actions or thoughts more easily. This can be due to brain changes or attempts to feel calmer.

- People may ask the same questions over and over again, or say the same things.
- People can get stuck on certain thoughts i.e. someone stealing from them.

Feelings about Mood Changes

Mood and Behaviour changes have a big impact on our lives.

These changes often cause difficulties with other people. This can make us feel upset more easily.

Here are some common feelings:

Confusion

Often other people will act differently with us because of changes in how we behave. These changes in how others act can be confusing.

- Losing our temper and shouting at others can happen more easily after brain injury. This can make other people feel scared or upset, and so they might avoid us.

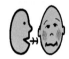

- Directly saying what we mean without thinking can make others uncomfortable. We might feel misunderstood or confused about this.

Anxiety

Changes after brain injury can make us feel more vulnerable and worried. Brain injury can make it difficult to control feelings of anxiety

- Feelings and worries can seem stronger and more difficult to manage after brain injury.
- It can be more difficult to feel reassured by others

Frustration and Anger

Difficulties with mood and behaviour can make us feel angry or frustrated with ourselves or other people

- When we find it difficult to stop ourselves from doing something that is not helpful (like losing our temper) it can be frustrating.

- We can become angry at other people when they act differently towards us, for example if they seem to be uncomfortable or fed up.

Feeling misunderstood or not valued

Mood and behaviour changes after brain injury can mean we feel misunderstood.

When other people act differently with us, we can feel like they do not care or are not listening. This may lead to us behaving differently:

- Shouting and getting angry when we need something can mean that other people do not help us
- Asking the same questions again and again is understandable when we feel unable to manage our anxiety by ourselves; but it is not always helpful if other people stop listening because they have answered the questions before.

Coping with Mood Changes

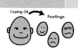

Mood and Behaviour changes after brain injury are common; however people do cope well with these. Here are some things people find help them cope:

Do things you enjoy!

Feeling happier with your life in general can help you stay calm and manage your emotions. For example:

- Listening to music or watching television

- Spending time with other people, i.e. friends and family

Use strategies

There are many skills you can learn to help you manage your emotions and behaviour.

- When you start getting angry, STOP and give yourself time to calm down

- When you feel vulnerable and uncertain, write down information which is comforting

Ask Other People for Support

It might help if other people know you have a brain injury. This helps them make sense of your mood and behaviour changes. It is also useful to ask for help:

- If you are feeling upset or angry
- If you are confused about the way other people are treating you

Speak to Psychology

People do learn skills to help manage mood and behaviour changes. Psychology can help by:

- Providing strategies to manage behaviour & mood
- Help people understand what is going on for you
- Support you to feel happier & work towards goals

Session 7:
Lifestyle Changes after Brain Injury

This session includes:

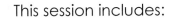

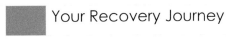 Your Recovery Journey

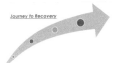

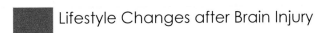 Lifestyle Changes after Brain Injury

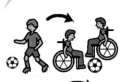

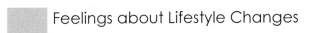 Feelings about Lifestyle Changes

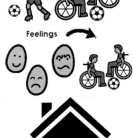

What can help after I leave?

Your Recovery Journey

Rehabilitation is to help you recover from brain injury. The goal of rehabilitation is to get you, as much as possible, back to your pre-injury self.

Recovery Journeys

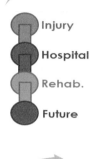

Recovery from brain injury is like a journey:

- Your brain injury marks the start of the journey
- Next, most people spend time in hospital
- When people are ready, they sometimes move to a rehabilitation unit
- The journey will continue after leaving...

Every person has a different "Recovery Journey".

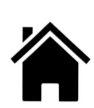

- Some people make almost a complete recovery
- Some people have difficulties that remain even after months of rehabilitation
- Other people continue to have difficulties and may find it difficult to live independently

Life After Hospital

Different people will take different paths.

Some people will:

- Go back to their homes
- Move somewhere else which is better suited to their needs
- Continue in rehabilitation somewhere else

Lifestyle Changes after Brain Injury

Reclaiming your life

Some people find that their lifestyle is different once they leave rehabilitation.

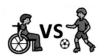

Most of the time, this just means that there are things you need to do to adjust to these differences

Some common differences are:

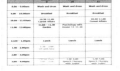

Structure: Rehabilitation is very structured. You have a timetable every day which you follow. After leaving rehab it can help to maintain this structure.

Socialising: Here people generally know about your difficulties and are good at communicating with people with brain injury. This may be more difficult after rehab – you may need to let other people know so that they can make adjustments

Work & hobbies: Many people want to get back to work and the things they enjoyed doing once they go back home. It can be helpful to consider what changes you need to make to continue doing the things you enjoy

Feelings about Lifestyle Changes

Lifestyle changes have a big impact on our lives, and this can stir up strong feelings.

People can be worried about the future, or have strong feelings about the changes they will have to make

Here are some common feelings:

Anxiety & Worry

Many people say that they are looking forward to getting back to their lives, but also feel a little bit worried about the way things have changed.

- Many people haven't seen their friends during rehab - they worry about how things will be.
- Some people worry about how well they will be able to do the things they used to do i.e. work.

These worries are understandable, but most people cope after rehabilitation.

Feeling Down

Some people really look forward to leaving rehab, but finding some things more difficult can make them feel sad or down

It is helpful to remember that there are many ways to continue doing the things you find important, and the things that you enjoy, with support and some changes

What can help after I leave?

After you leave Rehabilitation, there are many people that can help you to continue to recover:

Family and Friends

Having the support of your family and your friends can be really helpful.

- They can help with practical things, such as checking you are doing ok with everyday tasks
- They can give emotional support, and the chance for you to safely talk about difficulties

Health Services

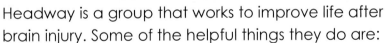

Once you leave rehab, you can still access health services in your local area. For example:

- Your GP
- Community therapists

Social Services

Social services will help you to get the care you need. For some people, this might be:

- Arranging a place for you to live that is suitable
- A Care Package which pays for carers to visit you at home

Charities and Support Groups

Headway is a group that works to improve life after brain injury. Some of the helpful things they do are:

- Support Groups
- Vocational Rehabilitation

Session 8:
My Goals for the Future

This session includes:

  Reviewing My Goals

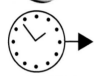 Moving towards My Future Goals

 UBI Group Summary

Reviewing My Goals

 You made some goals at the beginning of UBI Group. This was done in Session 1. Let's take a look at them:

 Short Term Goals

_____

_____

What progress have you made so far?

_____

 Medium Term Goals

_____

_____

What progress have you made so far?

_____

 Long Term Goals

_____

_____

What progress have you made so far?

_____

Look back over your goals and the progress you have made so far. What goals are still important?

_____

_____

What are your goals for when you leave Rehab?

1. _____

2. _____

3. _____

Moving Towards My Future Goals

Some goals for the future can seem difficult.
It helps to break these goals down to make the steps more manageable.

1. **Goal 1:**

What steps do I need to take to achieve this?

_____

_____

Goal 2:

What steps do I need to take to achieve this?

_____

_____

3. **Goal 3:**

What steps do I need to take to achieve this?

_____

_____

_____

UBI Group Summary

1. Introduction to the group.

This was the first group. We introduced the group, and talked about your goals.

2. The brain and brain injury

We gave you some information about the brain. We then talked about the effects of brain injury. You wrote about your own brain injury.

3. Rehabilitation

We talked with a therapist from Physiotherapy, Occupational Therapy, Speech and Language Therapy and Psychology about how each discipline helps you recover from your brain injury.

4. Physical changes after brain injury

We talked about the physical difficulties people have after brain injury. We talked about how these might make us feel, and how we can cope with them.

5. Thinking changes after brain injury

We talked about the thinking difficulties people have after brain injury. We talked about how these might make us feel, and how we can cope with them.

6. Mood changes after brain injury

We talked about the mood and behaviour difficulties people have after brain injury. We talked about how these changes might make us feel, and how we can cope with them.

7. Lifestyle changes after brain injury

We talked about life after you leave hospital. We talked about who can help you after you leave rehab.

8. Goals for the Future

Today's session! We spoke about what your goals are currently and for once you've left rehab.

With thanks to:

Dr Kevin Tierney, Clinical Psychologist

Dr Tarick Ali, Clinical Psychologist

The Picture Communication Symbols ©1981–2016 by Mayer-Johnson LLC a Tobii Dynavox company.

All Rights Reserved Worldwide. Used with permission. Boardmaker® is a trademark of Mayer-Johnson LLC.

Dr Rebekah Jamieson-Craig

Index

For Product Safety Concerns and Information please contact our
EU representative GPSR@taylorandfrancis.com Taylor & Francis
Verlag GmbH, Kaufingerstraße 24, 80331 München, Germany